THE TRIGLYCERIDES DIET BIBLE

Beginners' Diet Plans To Lower Triglycerides And Improve Health, Along With Tips, Recipes, And Changes To Your Daily Life

CRUE GAGE

Table of Contents

Introductory

Triglycerides are a form of lipid (fat) that are present in the bloodstream. They are the most prevalent form of fat in the body and are a significant source of energy. Triglycerides are made up of three fatty acids that are linked by a glycerol backbone.

Excess calories are converted into triglycerides and stored in fat cells for future use when they exceed the body's requirements, particularly from carbohydrates and lipids. An elevated risk of heart disease and other health complications may be linked to elevated levels of triglycerides in the blood.

<u>**Managing triglyceride levels is important for several reasons:**</u>

• **Heart Health**: High triglyceride levels can contribute to the hardening and narrowing of arteries (atherosclerosis), increasing the risk of heart disease and stroke.

• **Metabolic Health**: Elevated triglycerides are often associated with conditions like metabolic syndrome, which can lead to type 2 diabetes and other health complications.

• **Fatty Liver Disease**: High triglyceride levels can contribute to fatty liver disease, which can affect liver function and lead to more serious liver conditions.

• **Overall Wellness**: Maintaining healthy triglyceride levels is part of a balanced lifestyle that includes proper diet, exercise, and weight management, contributing to overall health and well-being.

Regular monitoring and lifestyle adjustments, such as diet and exercise, can help keep triglyceride levels within a healthy range.

Causes Of High Levels

High triglyceride levels can be caused by various factors, including:

• **Obesity**: Excess body weight, especially around the abdomen, can lead to increased triglyceride levels.

• **Poor Diet**: A diet high in refined carbohydrates, sugars, and unhealthy fats (such as trans fats) can raise triglyceride levels.

• **Physical Inactivity**: Lack of regular exercise can contribute to higher triglycerides.

• **Excess Alcohol Consumption**: Drinking alcohol in excess can increase triglyceride levels.

• **Medical Conditions**: Conditions like diabetes, hypothyroidism, kidney disease, and liver disease can affect triglyceride levels.

• **Genetic Factors**: Some people may have a genetic predisposition to high triglycerides, known as familial hypertriglyceridemia.

• **Medications**: Certain medications, including steroids, diuretics, and some beta-blockers, can also contribute to elevated triglyceride levels.

Managing these risk factors through lifestyle changes and, if necessary, medical treatment can help lower triglyceride levels.

CHAPTER ONE
Health Risks Associated With High Triglycerides

High triglyceride levels are associated with several health risks, including:

• **Heart Disease**: Elevated triglycerides can contribute to the buildup of plaque in arteries, increasing the risk of heart attack and stroke.

• **Metabolic Syndrome**: High triglycerides are a component of metabolic syndrome, which increases the risk of diabetes, heart disease, and stroke.

• **Type 2 Diabetes**: High triglyceride levels can be linked to insulin resistance, which can lead to the development of type 2 diabetes.

• **Pancreatitis**: Very high triglyceride levels can cause inflammation of the pancreas, leading to pancreatitis, which can be a serious condition.

• **Fatty Liver Disease**: Elevated triglycerides can contribute to non-alcoholic fatty liver disease (NAFLD), which may progress to liver damage and cirrhosis.

• **Kidney Disease**: High triglyceride levels can be associated with kidney problems, particularly in individuals with diabetes.

Managing triglyceride levels is crucial for reducing these risks and promoting overall health.

Dietary Factors Influencing Triglycerides

Dietary factors play a significant role in influencing triglyceride levels. Key dietary influences include:

• **Refined Carbohydrates**: Foods high in refined sugars and white flour (like pastries, white bread, and sugary drinks) can raise triglyceride levels.

• **Saturated and Trans Fats**: Diets high in unhealthy fats, such as those found in fried foods, processed snacks, and some margarines, can contribute to elevated triglycerides.

• **Alcohol**: Excessive alcohol consumption can lead to increased triglyceride production by the liver.

• **High-Calorie Diets**: Consuming more calories than the body needs, particularly from fats and sugars, can result in elevated triglyceride levels.

• **Omega-3 Fatty Acids**: Foods rich in omega-3 fatty acids (such as fatty fish, flaxseeds, and walnuts) can help lower triglyceride levels.

• **Fiber**: A diet high in soluble fiber (found in oats, fruits, vegetables, and legumes) can help reduce triglyceride levels by improving lipid metabolism.

• **Portion Control**: Eating large portions can lead to excess calorie intake, which can raise triglyceride levels.

Adopting a balanced diet with a focus on whole foods, healthy fats, and regular meals can help manage triglyceride levels effectively.

Foods To Embrace & Foods To Avoid

Foods to Embrace:

- **Fatty Fish**: Salmon, mackerel, and sardines are high in omega-3 fatty acids, which can help lower triglyceride levels.

- **Nuts and Seeds**: Walnuts, flaxseeds, and chia seeds provide healthy fats and fiber.

- **Whole Grains**: Oats, brown rice, quinoa, and whole wheat products are rich in fiber, which can help manage triglycerides.

- **Fruits and Vegetables**: Berries, apples, leafy greens, and cruciferous vegetables are high in antioxidants and fiber.

- **Legumes**: Beans, lentils, and peas are excellent sources of protein and fiber without the unhealthy fats.

- **Healthy Fats**: Olive oil and avocado provide monounsaturated fats, which can be beneficial.

Foods to Avoid:

- **Sugary Foods and Beverages**: Soft drinks, candy, and pastries can spike triglyceride levels due to high sugar content.
- **Refined Carbohydrates**: White bread, white rice, and other processed grains can lead to increased triglycerides.
- **Trans Fats**: Found in some margarines, fried foods, and packaged snacks, these should be avoided as they can raise triglyceride levels.

- **Saturated Fats**: Limit intake of red meat, full-fat dairy products, and processed meats, which can contribute to high triglycerides.

- **Excessive Alcohol**: High alcohol consumption can significantly raise triglyceride levels.

- **High-Calorie Foods**: Foods that are calorie-dense and low in nutrients, like chips and fast food, can lead to weight gain and higher triglycerides.

Focusing on a balanced diet while limiting or avoiding unhealthy options can help manage triglyceride levels effectively.

Cooking Techniques For Heart Health

Here are some heart-healthy cooking techniques:

- **Grilling**: Cooking meats and vegetables on a grill can reduce fat and enhance flavor without added oils.

- **Baking and Roasting**: These methods use dry heat, allowing for less fat usage while retaining nutrients. Try baking fish, chicken, or vegetables.

- **Steaming**: Steaming vegetables preserves nutrients and flavor without adding unhealthy fats.

- **Sautéing**: Use a small amount of healthy oil (like olive oil) for sautéing rather than butter or lard. Add garlic and herbs for flavor.

- **Broiling**: This method cooks food quickly with high heat from above, helping to reduce fat while adding a nice texture.

- **Slow Cooking**: Using a slow cooker can allow for tender meats and flavorful dishes without needing excess fat.

- **Pressure Cooking**: This method cooks food quickly while preserving nutrients and often requires less fat.

- **Using Herbs and Spices**: Flavor dishes with herbs and spices instead of salt or fatty sauces to enhance taste without compromising heart health.

Incorporating these techniques can help you create delicious meals that support cardiovascular health.

One-Week Meal Plan For Lowering Triglycerides

Here's a simple one-week meal plan designed to help lower triglycerides:

<u>Day 1:</u>

- **Breakfast**: Oatmeal topped with berries and a sprinkle of flaxseeds.
- **Lunch**: Quinoa salad with black beans, corn, diced peppers, and lime vinaigrette.
- **Dinner**: Grilled salmon with steamed broccoli and brown rice.
- **Snack**: A small handful of walnuts.

<u>Day 2:</u>

- **Breakfast**: Greek yogurt with sliced almonds and honey.

- **Lunch**: Spinach salad with chickpeas, cherry tomatoes, and balsamic dressing.
- **Dinner**: Baked chicken breast with roasted sweet potatoes and asparagus.
- **Snack**: Sliced apple with almond butter.

Day 3:

- **Breakfast**: Smoothie with spinach, banana, and unsweetened almond milk.
- **Lunch**: Lentil soup with a side of whole-grain bread.
- **Dinner**: Stir-fried tofu with mixed vegetables and quinoa.
- **Snack**: Carrot sticks with hummus.

Day 4:

- **Breakfast**: Whole-grain toast with avocado and poached egg.
- **Lunch**: Turkey and avocado wrap with whole grain tortilla and mixed greens.
- **Dinner**: Baked cod with lemon, garlic, and steamed green beans.
- **Snack**: A small bowl of mixed berries.

Day 5:

- **Breakfast**: Chia seed pudding made with almond milk and topped with fresh fruit.
- **Lunch**: Farro salad with roasted vegetables and a lemon dressing.
- **Dinner**: Grilled shrimp tacos with cabbage slaw and avocado on corn tortillas.

- **Snack**: Celery sticks with peanut butter.

Day 6:

- **Breakfast**: Smoothie bowl with banana, spinach, and topped with nuts and seeds.
- **Lunch**: Quinoa and roasted beet salad with goat cheese and walnuts.
- **Dinner**: Stuffed bell peppers with ground turkey, brown rice, and spices.
- **Snack**: Air-popped popcorn (unsalted).

Day 7:

- **Breakfast**: Overnight oats with chia seeds, topped with sliced banana.

- **Lunch**: Vegetable and bean chili with a side of whole-grain crackers.

- **Dinner**: Baked chicken thighs with Brussels sprouts and sweet potato mash.

- **Snack**: Greek yogurt with a drizzle of honey.

Tips:

- Stay hydrated by drinking plenty of water.

- Adjust portion sizes based on your individual needs.

Feel free to swap meals or ingredients to suit your preferences while keeping the focus on heart-healthy options.

CHAPTER TWO
Breakfast Recipes

Here are a few heart-healthy breakfast recipes to help lower triglycerides:

1. Oatmeal with Berries and Flaxseeds:

Ingredients:

- 1 cup rolled oats
- 2 cups water or unsweetened almond milk
- 1/2 cup mixed berries (fresh or frozen)
- 1 tablespoon ground flaxseeds
- Honey or maple syrup (optional)

Instructions:

- In a saucepan, bring water or almond milk to a boil.

- Stir in oats and reduce heat to a simmer. Cook for about 5 minutes or until thickened.
- Top with berries and flaxseeds. Drizzle with honey or maple syrup if desired.

2. Avocado Toast with Poached Egg:

Ingredients:

- 1 slice whole-grain bread
- 1/2 ripe avocado
- 1 egg
- Salt and pepper to taste
- Red pepper flakes (optional)

Instructions:

- Toast the whole-grain bread.
- Mash the avocado and spread it on the toast. Season with salt and pepper.

- Poach the egg: bring water to a gentle simmer, crack the egg into a small bowl, and gently slide it into the water. Cook for 3-4 minutes, then remove with a slotted spoon.
- Place the poached egg on top of the avocado toast. Sprinkle with red pepper flakes if desired.

3. Chia Seed Pudding:

Ingredients:

- 1/4 cup chia seeds
- 1 cup unsweetened almond milk (or any milk of choice)
- 1 tablespoon honey or maple syrup (optional)
- Fresh fruit and nuts for topping

Instructions:

- In a bowl or jar, mix chia seeds and almond milk. Stir well to prevent clumping.
- Add honey or maple syrup if desired and mix again.
- Cover and refrigerate for at least 2 hours or overnight.
- Serve topped with fresh fruit and nuts.

4. Greek Yogurt Parfait

Ingredients:

- 1 cup plain Greek yogurt
- 1/2 cup mixed fresh fruit (e.g., berries, banana, apple)
- 1/4 cup granola (preferably low-sugar)

- 1 tablespoon chopped nuts or seeds

Instructions:

- In a glass or bowl, layer Greek yogurt, fresh fruit, and granola.
- Sprinkle chopped nuts or seeds on top.
- Enjoy immediately!

5. Smoothie Bowl:

Ingredients:

- 1 banana
- 1/2 cup spinach
- 1/2 cup unsweetened almond milk
- 1 tablespoon peanut butter (or nut butter of choice)
- Toppings: sliced fruit, nuts, seeds, and granola

Instructions:

- In a blender, combine banana, spinach, almond milk, and peanut butter. Blend until smooth.
- Pour into a bowl and top with your choice of sliced fruit, nuts, seeds, and granola.

These recipes are nutritious, delicious, and supportive of heart health!

Lunch Recipes

Here are some heart-healthy lunch recipes to help lower triglycerides:

1. Quinoa Salad with Black Beans and Corn:

Ingredients:

- 1 cup cooked quinoa

- 1 can black beans, rinsed and drained
- 1 cup corn (fresh, frozen, or canned)
- 1 red bell pepper, diced
- 1/4 cup red onion, diced
- Juice of 1 lime
- 2 tablespoons olive oil
- Salt and pepper to taste
- Fresh cilantro (optional)

Instructions:

- In a large bowl, combine quinoa, black beans, corn, bell pepper, and red onion.
- In a small bowl, whisk together lime juice, olive oil, salt, and pepper.

- Pour dressing over the salad and toss to combine. Garnish with cilantro if desired.

2. Spinach Salad with Chickpeas and Avocado:

Ingredients:

- 4 cups fresh spinach
- 1 can chickpeas, rinsed and drained
- 1 avocado, diced
- 1/2 cup cherry tomatoes, halved
- 1/4 cup feta cheese (optional)
- 2 tablespoons balsamic vinaigrette

Instructions:

- In a large bowl, combine spinach, chickpeas, avocado, cherry tomatoes, and feta.

- Drizzle with balsamic vinaigrette and toss gently to combine.

3. Lentil Soup:

Ingredients:

- 1 cup lentils (green or brown)
- 1 onion, chopped
- 2 carrots, diced
- 2 celery stalks, diced
- 3 garlic cloves, minced
- 1 can diced tomatoes
- 4 cups vegetable broth
- 1 teaspoon cumin
- Salt and pepper to taste
- Olive oil

Instructions:

- In a pot, heat olive oil over medium heat. Sauté onion, carrots, and celery until softened.

- Add garlic and cumin, cooking for
  another minute.
- Stir in lentils, diced tomatoes, and
  vegetable broth. Bring to a boil.

Reduce heat and simmer for about 30 minutes, or until lentils are tender. Season with salt and pepper.

4. Turkey and Avocado Wrap:

Ingredients:

- 1 whole-grain tortilla
- 3-4 slices turkey breast (preferably low-sodium)
- 1/2 avocado, sliced
- Mixed greens or spinach
- Sliced tomato
- Mustard or hummus (optional)

Instructions:

- Spread mustard or hummus on the tortilla if desired.
- Layer turkey, avocado, greens, and tomato on the tortilla.
- Roll tightly and slice in half. Serve with a side of fresh fruit or veggies.

5. Farro Salad with Roasted Vegetables:

Ingredients:

- 1 cup cooked farro
- 1 cup assorted roasted vegetables (zucchini, bell peppers, carrots, etc.)
- 1/4 cup crumbled feta cheese (optional)
- 2 tablespoons olive oil
- Juice of 1 lemon
- Salt and pepper to taste

Instructions:

- Preheat the oven to 400°F (200°C). Toss vegetables with olive oil, salt, and pepper, and roast for about 20-25 minutes until tender.

- In a bowl, combine cooked farro, roasted vegetables, feta cheese, and lemon juice. Toss to combine and serve warm or at room temperature.

These lunches are nutritious, flavorful, and great for heart health!

Dinner Recipes

Here are some heart-healthy dinner recipes to help lower triglycerides:

1. Grilled Salmon with Steamed Broccoli and Brown Rice:

Ingredients:

- 2 salmon fillets
- 1 tablespoon olive oil
- Lemon juice
- Salt and pepper
- 2 cups broccoli florets
- 1 cup cooked brown rice

Instructions:

- Preheat the grill or a grill pan over medium heat. Brush salmon fillets with olive oil, lemon juice, salt, and pepper.

- Grill salmon for about 4-5 minutes per side, or until cooked through.
- Steam broccoli until tender (about 5-7 minutes).
- Serve grilled salmon with steamed broccoli and a side of brown rice.

2. Baked Chicken Breast with Roasted Sweet Potatoes and Asparagus:

Ingredients:

- 2 boneless, skinless chicken breasts
- 1 tablespoon olive oil
- 1 teaspoon paprika
- Salt and pepper
- 2 sweet potatoes, cubed
- 1 bunch asparagus, trimmed

Instructions:

- Preheat the oven to 400°F (200°C).

- Toss sweet potatoes with olive oil, paprika, salt, and pepper, and spread on a baking sheet.
- Bake sweet potatoes for 20 minutes, then add asparagus to the sheet and place chicken breasts seasoned with salt and pepper.
- Bake for an additional 20-25 minutes or until chicken is cooked through and vegetables are tender.

3.   Stir-Fried   Tofu   with   Mixed Vegetables:

Ingredients:

- 14 oz firm tofu, cubed
- 2 tablespoons soy sauce (low-sodium)
- 1 tablespoon olive oil or sesame oil

- 2 cups mixed vegetables (bell peppers, broccoli, snap peas, carrots)
- 2 cloves garlic, minced
- 1 teaspoon ginger, minced
- Cooked brown rice or quinoa (for serving)

Instructions:

- Heat oil in a large skillet over medium heat. Add cubed tofu and cook until golden brown, about 5-7 minutes. Remove and set aside.
- In the same skillet, add garlic and ginger, sautéing for about 1 minute.
- Add mixed vegetables and stir-fry until tender-crisp, about 5-7 minutes.

- Return tofu to the skillet and add soy sauce, cooking for an additional 2-3 minutes.
- Serve over brown rice or quinoa.

4. Stuffed Bell Peppers with Ground Turkey and Brown Rice:

Ingredients:

- 4 bell peppers, tops cut off and seeds removed
- 1 pound ground turkey (or lean beef)
- 1 cup cooked brown rice
- 1 can diced tomatoes
- 1 teaspoon Italian seasoning
- Salt and pepper
- Grated cheese (optional, for topping)

Instructions:

- Preheat the oven to 375°F (190°C).
- In a skillet, cook ground turkey over medium heat until browned. Add diced tomatoes, cooked rice, Italian seasoning, salt, and pepper. Mix well.
- Stuff each bell pepper with the turkey mixture and place in a baking dish. Top with cheese if desired.
- Cover with foil and bake for 25-30 minutes, then uncover and bake for an additional 10 minutes.

5. Baked Cod with Lemon and Garlic:

Ingredients:

- 2 cod fillets
- 2 tablespoons olive oil

- Juice of 1 lemon

- 2 cloves garlic, minced

- Salt and pepper

- Fresh parsley for garnish (optional)

Instructions:

- Preheat the oven to 400°F (200°C).

- In a baking dish, place cod fillets and drizzle with olive oil, lemon juice, garlic, salt, and pepper.

- Bake for 15-20 minutes or until the fish flakes easily with a fork.

- Garnish with fresh parsley before serving. Pair with steamed vegetables or a side salad.

These dinner recipes are not only delicious but also support heart health!

Here are some heart-healthy snack and dessert recipes to help lower triglycerides:

Snacks

1. Veggies and Hummus:

Ingredients:

- Assorted raw vegetables (carrots, celery, bell peppers, cucumber)
- 1 cup hummus (store-bought or homemade)

Instructions:

- Wash and cut the vegetables into sticks or bite-sized pieces.
- Serve with hummus for dipping.

2. Apple Slices with Almond Butter:

Ingredients:

- 1 apple, sliced
- 2 tablespoons almond butter (or peanut butter)

Instructions:

- Slice the apple and serve with almond butter for dipping.

3. Greek Yogurt with Honey and Walnuts:

Ingredients:

- 1 cup plain Greek yogurt
- 1 tablespoon honey
- 2 tablespoons chopped walnuts

Instructions:

- In a bowl, combine Greek yogurt with honey and top with chopped walnuts.

4. Popcorn (Air-Popped):

Ingredients:

- 1/4 cup popcorn kernels (air-popped)
- Olive oil or seasoning (optional)

Instructions:

- Pop the kernels in an air popper.
- Lightly drizzle with olive oil or sprinkle with your favorite seasoning (like nutritional yeast or a pinch of salt).

<u>**Desserts**</u>

1. Chia Seed Pudding:

Ingredients:

- 1/4 cup chia seeds
- 1 cup unsweetened almond milk (or any milk of choice)
- 1 tablespoon honey or maple syrup (optional)
- Fresh fruit for topping

Instructions:

- In a bowl or jar, mix chia seeds and almond milk. Stir well to prevent clumping.
- Add honey or maple syrup if desired, and mix again.
- Cover and refrigerate for at least 2 hours or overnight. Serve topped with fresh fruit.

2. *Banana Oatmeal Cookies:*

Ingredients:

- 2 ripe bananas, mashed
- 1 cup rolled oats
- 1/2 teaspoon cinnamon
- Optional: dark chocolate chips or nuts

Instructions:

- Preheat the oven to 350°F (175°C).
- In a bowl, mix mashed bananas, oats, and cinnamon. Stir in chocolate chips or nuts if using.
- Drop spoonfuls of the mixture onto a baking sheet lined with parchment paper.
- Bake for 12-15 minutes until set. Allow to cool before serving.

3. Baked Apples

Ingredients:

- 4 apples, cored
- 1/4 cup rolled oats
- 1/4 cup walnuts, chopped
- 1 tablespoon honey or maple syrup
- 1 teaspoon cinnamon

Instructions:

- Preheat the oven to 350°F (175°C).
- In a bowl, mix oats, walnuts, honey, and cinnamon.
- Stuff the mixture into the cored apples.
- Place apples in a baking dish with a bit of water at the bottom and bake for 20-25 minutes until tender.

These snacks and desserts are delicious, nutritious, and supportive of heart health! Enjoy!

Lifestyle Modifications

Here are some effective lifestyle modifications to help lower triglyceride levels and promote overall heart health:

1. Healthy Diet:

- **Focus on Whole Foods**: Emphasize fruits, vegetables, whole grains, lean proteins, and healthy fats.
- **Limit Sugar Intake**: Reduce consumption of sugary foods and beverages.
- **Choose Healthy Fats**: Opt for unsaturated fats (olive oil, avocados, nuts) instead of saturated and trans fats.

- **Increase Fiber**: Incorporate more soluble fiber through foods like oats, beans, and fruits.

2. Regular Physical Activity:

- **Aim for 150 Minutes**: Engage in moderate-intensity aerobic exercise (like brisk walking) for at least 150 minutes per week.
- **Include Strength Training**: Incorporate strength training exercises at least twice a week.

3. Maintain a Healthy Weight:

- **Weight Loss**: If overweight, losing even a small percentage of body weight (5-10%) can help lower triglyceride levels.

- **Monitor Portion Sizes**: Be mindful of portion sizes to avoid overeating.

4. Limit Alcohol Consumption:

• **Drink in Moderation**: If you consume alcohol, do so in moderation (up to one drink per day for women and two for men).

5. Quit Smoking:

• **Avoid Tobacco**: If you smoke, seek help to quit. Non-smokers should avoid exposure to secondhand smoke.

6. Manage Stress

• **Practice Stress-Reduction Techniques**: Engage in activities like yoga, meditation, deep breathing, or hobbies that you enjoy.

7. Get Enough Sleep:

• **Aim for 7-9 Hours**: Prioritize quality sleep each night, as poor sleep can affect metabolic health.

8. Regular Health Check-ups:

• **Monitor Triglyceride Levels**: Regular check-ups with your healthcare provider can help track progress and make necessary adjustments.

Incorporating these lifestyle modifications can lead to significant improvements in triglyceride levels and overall heart health.

Long-Term Strategies For Maintaining Healthy Triglyceride Levels

Maintaining healthy triglyceride levels over the long term involves consistent lifestyle choices. Here are some effective strategies:

1. Adopt a Balanced Diet:

• **Focus on Nutrient-Dense Foods**: Prioritize whole foods like fruits, vegetables, whole grains, lean proteins, and healthy fats.

• **Limit Processed Foods**: Avoid foods high in sugar, refined carbohydrates, and unhealthy fats.

2. Stay Physically Active:

• **Make Exercise a Habit**: Aim for at least 150 minutes of moderate aerobic exercise each week, along with strength training exercises.

• **Incorporate Movement**: Look for opportunities to be active throughout the day (e.g., walking, taking the stairs).

3. Monitor Weight:

• **Maintain a Healthy Weight**: Keep track of your weight and make adjustments as necessary. Aim for gradual, sustainable weight loss if overweight.

4. Limit Alcohol Intake:

• **Drink in Moderation**: If you drink, do so in moderation to avoid increases in triglyceride levels.

5. Manage Stress Effectively:

• **Practice Stress Management Techniques**: Incorporate practices such as meditation, yoga, deep breathing, or mindfulness to reduce stress levels.

6. Get Regular Health Check-Ups

• **Monitor Lipid Levels**: Have regular check-ups to monitor your triglyceride levels and overall cardiovascular health.

• **Discuss Medications if Necessary**: Talk to your healthcare provider about any medications that may be needed to manage triglycerides.

7. Stay Hydrated:

• **Drink Plenty of Water**: Staying hydrated can support overall metabolic health and help manage weight.

8. Educate Yourself:

• **Stay Informed**: Keep learning about nutrition and health to make informed choices that support heart health.

9. Build a Support System:

• **Engage Family and Friends**: Surround yourself with supportive people who encourage healthy habits.

In the long term, it is possible to maintain healthy triglyceride levels and improve your overall cardiovascular health by consistently implementing these strategies.

Conclusion

It is essential to maintain healthy triglyceride levels in order to reduce the risk of cardiovascular disease and promote overall cardiac health.

By incorporating stress-reduction techniques, managing weight, engaging in regular physical activity, and adopting a balanced diet rich in whole foods, you can make substantial progress in enhancing your triglyceride levels. Long-term success necessitates consistent check-ups and education regarding cardiovascular health.

It is important to bear in mind that modest, sustainable lifestyle modifications can result in substantial health advantages over time.

By adhering to these strategies, you can foster improved health and well-being for the long term.

THE END